How Could You Let This Happen?

By

Rebecca McGrue

All of the person's names contained within this book are fictitious. Any resemblance to any persons, either living or dead, is entirely coincidental.

To my wonderful husband, Charles: You encouraged me to do this project, and supported me every step of the way. You have been such a precious gift from God.

Forward

Seven years have passed since I escaped my first marriage. I spent 16 years in an emotionally and physically abusive relationship. I was not beaten black and blue every day, so I spent the majority of those years unaware of what was happening to me. I never considered I was being beaten down emotionally. My life drastically changed once I recognized there was nothing wrong with me, and I deserved to be happy; however, my path to happiness and healing was a challenge. I endured a great deal of stress and misery before I was able to truly set myself free.

Although my ex-husband has never been formally diagnosed, that I am aware of, he meets the criteria for Narcissistic Personality Disorder. According to the Diagnostic and Statistical Manual of Mental Disorders, individuals with this disorder have: an inflated sense of self, lack of empathy for others, a sense of entitlement, jealousy of others, require excessive admiration, are manipulative, take advantage of others, and are unwilling take responsibility for their actions.

The purpose of this book is to disclose my experiences in the hopes of educating people on the traits of someone who meets the criteria for Narcissistic Personality Disorder; so they can identify it, and not succumb to what I went through. In other words, warning anyone who may be in a relationship with a narcissist. I will focus on this by laying out the development of an unhealthy relationship Our minds are not wired for introspection; therefore, it can be very difficult to recognize abuse when it is present in our relationships. At the time, I was unable to explain that to my mother when she asked me, "How could you let this happen?"

I was not a prisoner in the relationship, and take full responsibility for staying in it as long as I did. One of the reasons I stayed was because I was unaware of the abuse; I

5

normalized it. I also struggled with making my daughter a product of a divorce. I did not want to hurt her even though I was very unhappy. The abuse in my marriage significantly amplified when my daughter was six years old. It was then when I finally realized we were exposing her to a very unhealthy relationship. At that point I knew I had to get out.

One

My formative years took place in central California. I was the youngest child of three daughters. We were a middle- classed, Mexican family, but we did not have the traditional Mexican household. My parents never spoke Spanish to us, nor were we exposed to Mexican culture. They wanted us to identify with people, not a nationality. They were also extremely protective of all of us, and were very loving. I was more outgoing than my older sisters, Marie and Elizabeth. I was the one who didn't hesitate to speak her mind. My mother labeled me, "Becca the mouth." Whereas my father called me, "his little bitch." They of course did not mean to be hurtful with the nicknames; however, I wish my outspokenness was encouraged, instead of ridiculed.

My mother took very good care of us. My father was good to us as well; however, he often travelled during his career, and was gone a lot. My mom was a PTA   mom, brownie troop leader, and made most of our clothes. She stopped participating in those activities when I came along. I didn't get the same mother my siblings did, because she chose to go back to work when I started school. I don't feel I was offered or exposed to the same activities as my sisters. I think she figured I didn't need her as much. My mother never played with any of her children either. She stated she didn't know how. As a result, I often felt lonely, and created an imaginary friend.

We were extremely sheltered! My mother never taught us to cook because she didn't want us in her kitchen. I was 17 years old before learning to wash my own clothes. Our parents did not teach us how to use a check book either. I'm not sure why I wasn't taught to be self-sufficient at an earlier age. I think my mom was used to taking care of all of us; maybe her mother did all of these things for her until she left home. I taught myself to be independent.

For many reasons I remember feeling insignificant while growing up. My mother was the type of parent when asked for an explanation about something, would respond with, "Because I said so." I feel that ultimately made me a better mother to my daughter, because I would never want her to feel her questions didn't matter. I am very considerate in regards to her feelings. My parents never spanked us, but if I did misbehave, my mother grabbed me by the arm, shook and scolded me as she walked me to my room. It was humiliating. As an adult, I overheard her describe that scenario to other people, as she laughed about it.

My maternal grandmother and I used to be very close. She was childlike, and usually disclosed information to me which a child should not be subjected. For example, she informed me at a very young age the middle child, Elizabeth, was my mom and dad's favorite. Elizabeth suffered from anxiety and depression. My parents considered her a very sensitive and special child, and wanted us to tip-toe around her- don't upset her! They made excuses for anything negative she did, and they still do. I was expected to know better if I misbehaved. Marie was ten years older than I am, and I don't recall her ever getting into trouble.

One of the most hurtful memories I have as a child occurred at age five. My immediate family accused me of lying in order to get attention. Unfortunately, my family has a long history of denial and keeping secrets. This has caused a great deal of unnecessary anguish. One of the major secrets involved something that happened in our house when I was a year old. We had a poltergeist, for lack of a better explanation. Objects moved around in our house over the course of a year. Many items came to me, and ended up in my crib or playpen. It's as if the energy that occupied our home wanted to entertain me. The reason I know these things truly did happen is because these events occurred again when I was 16 years old, and I witnessed them. My grandmother was fascinated by the events that occurred when I was a baby. She decided to tell me all about it when I was five years old. She was extremely animated when she spoke.

She stated I was magic, and when I was a baby I used to make things fly. She told me not to mention my knowledge of this to my parents. That doesn't last very long when you are five years old. I thought it was wrong to keep secrets from my parents, so I told them the story my grandmother told me. They were furious, and I got in trouble for mentioning it. My mother accused me of lying and wanting attention. My two older sisters are five and ten years older than I am. So, they were old enough to remember the events that took place in the house. They also shared our mother's disgust, and accused me of wanting attention. I remember feeling so ashamed of myself, yet confused because I was merely repeating what I was   told.

Again, unnecessary anguish was caused just because my family wanted to keep certain things hidden.

For some reason, many Mexican families like to scare their children. I learned this happened to my grandmother, her siblings, and both my parents. Unfortunately, this was the part of the Mexican culture my parents exposed to us. The devil (El Cucuy) was always used as a scare tactic. I have been afraid of the dark my entire life. I used to put lights on all over the house when walking from one room to the next in the evening. One night my father encouraged me to be brave, and to do so without putting on a bunch of lights. I gathered up my strength, and did as he asked. My father yelled out, "the devil is going to get you," when I was in the middle of crossing one of the bedrooms. I screamed with fear, and he laughed at me. I never understood how this amused adults, or why anyone would want to scare their child.

My mother did the same thing to me when she wanted me to go to sleep. I used to share a bedroom with Elizabeth, and usually told jokes and stories to her long after we were supposed to be asleep. My mom came to our room several times, and warned me to settle down for the night. Her last attempt involved telling me the devil was going to come through my window and get me if I didn't go to sleep. I am 42 years old and I still struggle with being in the dark because of those incidents.

I do have to add there were a lot of happy moments while growing up. There were birthday parties, surprises, family vacations, and many times I did feel special. I wrote a play when I was about six years old, and my dad performed in it with me at the house. It meant so much to me that he took the time to dress up in a suit at my request, and follow my script. I always knew my parents loved me. I also knew they would never intentionally hurt me. They parented how they knew best.

Unfortunately, I suffered a lot of emotional grief because of our family's dysfunctions. Do I place blame on my family for my decisions or who I became? I certainly do not! I disclosed all of this as a means of understanding the world in which I grew up. However, I don't feel I was taught to value myself.

Two

I first met Danny through a friend when I was 16 years old. He was 18 at the time. My friend, Mabel was dating his friend, Raymond. One evening I was visiting her when Raymond came to the house. He brought Danny along as well. Danny was quiet and very polite. I didn't have any interest in him as I wasn't attracted to him at all. He was awkwardly tall and had a chunky face. I spoke to him to be polite. After chatting with him that evening I felt he was a really nice guy. He asked for my number, and I gave it to him. We talked a few times on the phone. I felt he was very easy to talk to, and I enjoyed our conversations. I agreed to let him take me out. We went to the movies the following week. He was a perfect gentleman, and we had a nice time.

He was even funny. Ironically, I felt he was too nice. He also didn't appear to be very outgoing, and was a little shy. Most of the guys I had previously dated were extroverted and fun. I didn't answer his calls anymore after our first date. How I wish I would have left well enough alone.

I saw Danny again when I was 19 years old. I was working at the Disney Store in our local mall. He passed through with his girlfriend and their infant daughter. My first thought was, "I dodged a bullet; he has a baby now." He came back into the store a month later to see me, and was alone. We began to chat, and he stated he and his daughter's mother were no longer together. I didn't find out until late in our marriage that was a lie. Danny appeared to be a very nice person. He seemed like he was the type of guy you could tell anything to, and a great friend.

We became close very quickly. He came to my house to visit me all the time, and I loved the attention. He was not only my boyfriend, but a close friend. I shared everything with him about my life, fears, insecurities, and what bothered me about my family. I told him I felt trapped sometimes because my parents were so strict with me. He began to tell me that I deserved respect too, and my parents weren't giving it to me. Danny said they treated me like a baby, and encouraged me to rebel against them. He told me how he understood my frustrations and he was on my side, as if it was us against them. What I didn't realize at the time is he was grooming me to completely trust him and all of his ideas.

Danny was also very jealous of me. I had parents who cared about me enough to place rules on me and showed an interest in my life. Danny didn't even live with his parents. They were divorced when he was a young boy, and his mother remarried. She lived in a town about an hour and half away with his step-father. His father lived in his work studio, and was an alcoholic who used to abuse Danny's mother and sister. Danny lived with his   maternal grandmother. He had minimal to no contact with his father, and described his mother as very selfish.

I don't know a great deal about Danny's childhood; however, the few incidents I was told of were disturbing. He told me his father used to beat his older sister because she was a girl. When his sister was a teenager, she and their father threw phones and various objects at each other when they got into a dispute. His aunt Carmen confirmed this as well. Danny also witnessed his father slamming the back door on his mother's hands when she tried to leave somewhere he didn't want her to go. The door took off part of her finger.

His mother suffered from depression. I feel her depression was the reason Danny never felt nurtured by her. His mother disclosed to me that she and Danny's father both had full- time jobs; yet, she was expected to make a five course meal with homemade tortillas every night. She never told me what would happen otherwise. Danny was never taught to respect women, because his male role model was so demanding and abusive. I cannot recall what age Danny was when his parents finally divorced, but I believe he was in junior high.

Danny was in high school when his mother married his step-father, Brad. Brad had two sons from a previous marriage, and felt Danny was a bad influence on them, considering Danny often got in trouble at school. Danny's mother told me she didn't know what to do when her new husband suggested Danny live elsewhere. So, she shared her predicament with Danny. That always angered me that a mother expressed to her son how she felt she had to choose between them. That was a worry he never should have had to endure. His mother ultimately sent him to live with his sister who was renting an apartment at the time. His mother supported him financially.

Danny said his sister always kept the temperature in the apartment freezing, and she was angry all the time.

After a couple of years he went to live with his maternal grandmother. That is pretty much all I know about his formative years.

My parents never liked Danny. They didn't want me to date a single dad who didn't appear to have any ambition to be successful in life. My father expressed a great amount of disgust in him for failing to financially support his baby. He was a dishwasher for a barbeque restaurant when we started dating. He soon quit after he got into an argument with the owner. He claimed she never liked him, and treated him unfairly. It took me years to realize that he felt nothing was ever his fault. According to him, someone always had it in for him, or he was given a bad deal. He usually did not take ownership for anything he did. My parents warned me about him. Everyone I knew thought he was a loser, and was too possessive of me. All I saw was this fun guy who emotionally supported me when I felt so alone.

We had a lot of fun together as well. We hung out with mutual friends, went to the movies, travelled out of town to the beach (which I always paid for), and attended parties together. We had sex very early in our relationship, and engaged in intercourse almost every time we saw each other. When I was 19 he took me to Ensenada, Mexico to dance and have fun in the bars. He used to loan me his truck while he was at work, and said to go have fun with my friends. It was an exciting time for me because I had never been in a relationship where a guy showed me so much interest. I enjoyed the attention. Danny had this silly way about him, and I thought he was fun to be around. What else are you looking for in a guy when you are 19?

He also taught me how to drive a stick shift, and was very patient with me when doing so. If we went out together, he ran to his truck and sat in the passenger seat so I would have to practice driving. I used to get nervous, but he always asked me to try. We had many moments when it seemed as though he really cared about me.

The transition from my parent's control to Danny's control was swift. I used to ride my bike around town a great deal. That was my alone time which I enjoyed. I also loved the exercise. One afternoon Danny passed by my house, and saw me on my bike at a nearby convenience store. He approached me, and asked that I not go riding around town by myself. I assured him I had done so many times, and stayed in safe neighborhoods. He was relentless, and stated he was worried about me. It became an argument because I didn't agree with him. He told me, "You can go ahead and go but, it will cause problems between us." I allowed him to manipulate me, and I ended up going home. He proceeded to tell me how much he cared about me, and wanted to keep me safe. What I had showed him at that point was how much control he already had over me. That occurred during our first year together. Danny had two best friends, Raymond and Pete. They warned me about Danny's manipulative behavior from the very beginning. They stated he always tried to get what he wanted, and didn't consider other people's feelings. That angered Danny. He accused them of trying to sabotage our relationship because of jealousy.

Danny broke up with me one day because it frustrated him that I had a curfew. He stated, "I can't stand how your parents treat you. You'll always be under their thumb." I was 20 years old, but I had to follow my parent's rules since I lived with them. I wanted to prove to him that I was an adult. I wasn't about to lose a relationship because of my parents. We got back together and I started rebelling. I went out with him whenever I wanted, and distanced myself from my family. He also used to make fun of how I called my father, "Daddy." He mocked me and said, "Daddy" in a high pitched voice. He teased me about that throughout our entire relationship.

Part of a Narcissist's cycle is to nose-dive into a depression at times. Danny disclosed a great deal that hurt him during those periods, and he cried. He often stated he felt like he raised himself, because he always felt so alone. He also said his parents were very cruel when they scolded him as a child. He mentioned the relationship with his mother used to be fun-loving after his parents divorced. Apparently they joked around a lot and he loved it. That came to an end after his step-father came into the picture. Danny said his mother became prim and proper after marrying Brad. She told Danny that her new husband felt it was disrespectful to joke around with her as he did. He described an argument he had with his mother regarding her behavior towards him. He said he tried to explain to her how much he missed the fun times between the two of them but, she would not listen. He said he grabbed her by the neck, and pushed her up against the wall so she would listen to him. He wanted her to hear how horribly she was neglecting him. It did not occur to me how physically aggressive he was after hearing that story. I felt very sorry for him, and how desperately hurt he was about his life. He usually had a way of explaining something so his actions were justified.

Grandiosity is another characteristic of a Narcissist. Danny informed me many times throughout our relationship how he had a higher level of understanding than most people. He felt he had achieved an awareness that many people could only dream of possessing. This came from a man who has never read a book in his life. It appeared as though he felt he was intellectually above most people. That is the reason for his inability to admit being wrong. He disclosed to me that his mother had taken him to a counselor when he was younger. He felt he knew more than the counselor did, and enjoyed challenging her.

Danny had a desperate need to feel loved as well. Early on in our relationship he asked me if I loved him. I liked him a lot, but did not feel love for him yet. I was honest, and told him how I felt. He pressed the issue for days. "Are you sure you don't love me even just a little bit?" he asked. He definitely pressured me to say those three little words. So, I told him I loved him, and he was content. I had never met anyone who asked to be loved, nor did I know what to think about it. Now I understand that narcissist's need a great deal of love and admiration because of their fragile sense of self-worth.

One afternoon, I went to visit him while his family was having a yard sale. After it was over, everyone sat around the front yard and was talking. His mother was in town visiting that weekend as well. One of his cousins started talking about motorcycles. Danny stated how much he wanted one. He proceeded to blame his mother for never buying one for him. He became very angry and began to pout.

Danny said how messed up his mom was, because she knew how much he wanted one, and never bought one for him. The whole family became quiet, and it appeared as though we were all embarrassed for him. He made a fool of himself. Danny acted like a young child who was throwing a fit because he did not get what he wanted. He later told me he felt justified in his complaints, because his mother should have given him what he wanted since she fell short in being a good mother. His step-father had given him his old truck to use at that time. Ironically, he is now 43 years old and currently driving a different truck that his step-father gave him. He continuously shows a strong sense of entitlement.

Danny became quite comfortable with saying and doing anything with me during our first year together. That included making fun of me and "play fighting." He began to point out my many imperfections. He didn't like that I was flat-footed, and told me not to stand a certain way. He said it looked like my ankles were going to break. My ribs stuck out a little further than most people he knew, so he made fun of those as well. I can't forget Frankenstein head, either. Apparently, my forehead was not as flat as he felt it should be. He pointed out this bump, and encouraged me to cover it with my bangs. I was extremely self- conscience about my forehead, and kept my bangs until I met my current husband at age 37.

I expressed to Danny how much I disliked that he made fun of me. He said I was too sensitive, and he was just playing around. He was always "just playing around," and never took ownership for his actions. He also criticized my faith. I was raised as a Catholic, and Danny was raised in a non-denominational faith. He never went to church; however, he always made it a point to not only challenge my beliefs, but tell me they were wrong. Narcissists typically find faults in anyone who does not mirror their image. I was still trying to figure out who I was during that period. Being told there was so much wrong with me by someone who supposedly cared about me had a very deep impact.

Danny took me out to a park when he wanted to play fight. He kicked and punched me, and stated I was too much of a wimp, and needed to be toughened up. He usually started by trying to provoke me to chase him by slapping me on the back of the head. Of course I tried to defend myself, but always ended up with bruises all over my legs and arms. Danny used to laugh, and said we were just playing. I did not see this as abuse; however, I didn't like it and asked him to stop. He stopped when he felt I had enough, and said I was weak. It saddens me to remember how much I trusted him, and did not understand that I was being abused.

He also kicked me at a house party during our first year together. Everyone was sitting in a living room where we were laughing and joking with one another. I cannot specifically remember what it was that I said, but I was being playful and made a comment about Danny. He got up from the couch, and kicked me three times on the shin. It hurt so badly; I thought I was going to vomit. I was shocked and humiliated because everyone was staring at us. He proceeded to yell at me for being a bitch. The rest of the details are too foggy. All I remember is he never apologized, and stated I shouldn't have made fun of him. He blamed me for disrespecting him, and making him angry. I unintentionally embarrassed him. That's unacceptable to someone who thinks he's above everyone. I ended up blaming myself for the attack. I figured I was the one who instigated it.

Danny chose big rig truck driving as a profession. He was dyslexic, and used that as an excuse not to go to college. He stated he was only capable of driving because the job didn't require a lot of reading. Sometimes I rode with him when he went far away. He always wanted to include me with what he was doing. I didn't find out about the dyslexia until a couple of years after we were together. I tried to help him with it, and we went to the library to study a couple of times a week. I bought him a workbook, and he started to make progress. He stopped wanting my help after a couple of months. He stated he didn't have the patience for it, and blamed me for not making it fun enough for him. The truth was, he didn't like being challenged, and had to place blame on someone for rejecting the opportunity to learn.

One weekend Danny met a girl named, Vivienne through his friend Raymond. She was our age and lived on her own. Her parents had passed away, and she took care of her two younger sisters who weren't that much younger than she was. He spoke very highly of her for taking care of her siblings. Raymond was dating one of Vivienne's sisters. He used to take Danny with him to visit. Sound familiar? They spent a great deal of time visiting the girls, and I was very jealous. I asked why he couldn't take me with him. Danny ultimately told me that I wouldn't fit in with them. He stated that I acted "too white" to hang out with everyone at Vivienne's house. He said his time over there as perfectly innocent. He said they played Mexican music and danced. Many times he said they watched movies. One day he admitted taking Vivienne with him over night in the truck. He said that he took her just as a companion, and that he could tell her things I wouldn't understand.

I am not sure why I didn't leave him as I had plenty of other guys asking me out. I even went out on dates with different guys I had liked since high school; guys who were so much nicer, smarter, and more respectful than Danny. I think maybe it was a challenge to try to keep him at that point- some juvenile game? I was so insecure at that point. I felt I was lucky to be with him considering there was so much wrong with me. He ridiculed my body, clothes, decisions and beliefs. According to him, he needed to show me the right way to think. I also didn't want to be alone. He was a constant, even though he caused me so much pain. He eventually stopped hanging out with her, and we moved passed it. Things got better between us for a while.

We also had many issues with his daughter's mother, Melissa. She became very upset any time she saw us out together, and paged him to call her. If he did call her, he walked away from me, and did so privately. He used to take Melissa and his daughter for overnight trips to his mom's house in the next town. I was so naive! I never had a clue that he was seeing her as well. He told me it was a unique situation since he had a daughter with her, and I didn't understand he had to spend time with her as well as the baby. I usually ended up feeling guilty about mentioning my concerns about her behavior in regards to our relationship. He got angry any time I mentioned it, and said I was being selfish.

Danny manipulated both of us. Raymond broke Danny's confidence and warned me that he bragged about having both of us at his heels. It was ultimately dropped when Danny denied it.

There was a time when some male strippers came into town and performed at the local strip club. A few of my girlfriends invited me to go with them. I wanted to go as it had been a while since I participated in a girl's night out. My mother even told me to go and have fun because she felt I spent all my free time with Danny. I told Danny about it at the end of our date the weekend prior to the event. He told me he didn't want me to go. I felt he was being a hypocrite, because he had gone to the same club several times with his friends. I proceeded to tell him I was going, and wasn't doing anything wrong.

This turned into a fight. We were standing in my front yard, and I turned my back on him to go inside. That infuriated him, and he followed me to the front door. I made it inside, but he grabbed my arm to stop me. I yelled at him to let go of me, and tried closing the door on him. My mother was in the living room and saw this. Danny let go of my arm as soon as he saw her. She yelled at both of us for fighting. Instead of telling him to leave, she allowed him to come in so we could work it out. Danny calmed down very quickly in front of my mother. She left us alone, and we continued to discuss the matter. He ultimately told me he was upset because I didn't ask his permission to go. I was extremely disgusted by that. He ended up changing his attitude, and became very sweet with me. I allowed him to manipulate me into not going. We ended up spending the following weekend together as usual. My friends were put off by this as it was not the first time something like that had happened. They stopped inviting me out with them after that incident.

It was very difficult to write the contents of our first couple of years together. What I have described so far   are examples of emotional and physical abuse. Emotional abuse takes many forms, and is considered the following: Abusive Expectations, Aggressing, and Verbal Assaults. Abusive Expectations occurs when an individual places unreasonable demands on you, and expects you to drop everything to cater to their needs. That was often the case with Danny. His needs were more important than mine. Aggressing is when an individual uses name-calling, accuses, blames, threatens or orders you around. Verbal Assaults include berating, belittling, criticizing, screaming, excessive blaming, sarcasm and humiliation. I endured all of this within our first year together. It sickens me to remember and recognize what I tolerated.

I've tried not to judge myself, because so many have done that for me. I have never had a vindictive or cruel mind. That is why it was so inconceivable to me that someone I chose to be with would intentionally hurt me.

Three

I moved in with Danny when I was 22 years old. My parents owned a duplex and we rented one of the apartments from them. My mother had always talked about how she couldn't wait until all of her kids moved out. I thought this was the perfect opportunity to escape my parent's control, and to be on my own with Danny. We had a lot of fun. We had friends over and we went out all of the time. He liked taking me out to big steak dinners in the next town. It was nice doing what I wanted to do. We also used to have squirt gun fights when we got home from work. We were two big kids living on our own.

I was going to a junior college at that time, and taking classes to be a social worker. I stopped going to school by the end of our first year in our apartment. I couldn't afford classes on my own anymore, and Danny was against the profession. He stated I would have been working with scum if I were to become a social worker, and felt I shouldn't be around low-class people. There were also many times throughout our relationship he told me I would never make a good therapist. I had told him I was interested in that profession. He often said I didn't understand things, and was too ditsy. He was persistent in trying to break down my sense of self, and unknowingly, I allowed him to succeed.

I still didn't recognize that he continued to bully me. One afternoon I was taking a hot shower. Danny came into the bathroom, reached over the shower rod, and poured a bucket of cold water on me. I almost went into shock. I was momentarily confused, and became off-balance. I screamed once I realized what happened. Danny started laughing, and told me to lighten up. A couple of different times he held my nose and mouth shut when I was asleep to see how long I could go without air before waking up. He laughed hysterically each time I woke up gasping for air.

According to him, it was all in the name of fun. He teased me, and said I was dumb because I didn't realize in my sleep that I couldn't breathe for a long time. Many things about his "playfulness" annoyed me; however, I allowed him to convince me that he was not doing anything wrong. I was always told that I was too sensitive if something bothered me. I guess eventually I got tired of defending myself and started to believe him.

I began to experience emotional difficulties after we lived together for a few months. I often felt very sad, angry and frustrated. I was growing tired of his constant contradictions, and had a bad attitude a great deal of the time. I also felt irritable and sad when it came to issues he was unwilling to resolve. Nothing between us was ever resolved. I learned that if I had a problem with the way things were, I needed to keep quiet about it, as he would blame me or find a reason it was ok. For example, Danny expected me to call him and let him know if I was going to be late from work. Then he would decide if it was a necessary reason. If not, I would have to skip what I planned, and come home anyway. The same did not apply for him. Danny came and went as he pleased, and paid no consideration to the way I felt. I wasn't sure why I always had an attitude and was easily irritated. Danny felt I had issues.

I didn't want to give up, even though I was unhappy with the way things were between us. I felt a relationship took work, and it was never going to be perfect; however, I was the only one who was willing to put forth any effort. Danny felt everything should work out around his needs.

He asked me to marry him despite all of our arguing. I think I felt his proposal proved his feelings for me. I was very excited and we immediately started planning a wedding. I didn't take any of our past issues into consideration before agreeing to marry him. I was only 23 years old at the time, and in love with the concept of being married. The whole idea of having a big wedding was exciting as well. I chose to get married for all of the wrong reasons. I had a beautiful dress picked out, and asked my best friend and sisters to be bride's maids. It was definitely an exciting time. My parents were supportive, and my dad reserved a hall for the wedding. Danny's mother and step-father were very nice to me, and looked forward to the event as well.

Alicia is Danny's older sister. She had her wedding during that time. She didn't speak to their father, so she asked Danny to give her away. The two of them never got along either, but Danny was all she had. Alicia was close to Melissa, and had her and Danny's daughter, Ann in the wedding. Danny did not allow Melissa to bring her boyfriend to the event. He argued it was disrespectful towards him, and stated he wanted to be the center of Ann's attention. He didn't want to have to share her with her boyfriend. I was uncomfortable about his concern over Melissa's boyfriend, and felt his thought process was childish. But, I kept it to myself. I did have an opportunity to meet a great deal of the family. Everyone was very nice to me. I was never very comfortable around them, but at the time I enjoyed being accepted by everyone. Like my own family, they had their dysfunctions. They were not a very loving, and seemed to place a great deal of importance on material items.

Danny became very ill with Valley Fever a couple of months after his sister's wedding. This is a disease caused by a fungus that gets into your body through your lungs. This fungus lives in the soil and is typically released into the air as crops are plowed. We lived in a farm town. And the small towns surrounding ours were all farm towns. Many individuals who lived in the area tested positive for the disease, but never developed any symptoms. Symptoms are flu-like and range from mild to severe. The disease can also be life threatening. Danny's case was severe, and it spread to his lymph nodes. He ended up on disability because he could no longer drive. He was very weak, pale and lost a great deal of weight. Neither one of us handled the stress very well. We fought a lot as money was tight, and the uncertainty of his health weighed heavily on us. We were unable to handle the stress because our relationship lacked a strong foundation, and had always been very turbulent. The doctor who treated Danny suggested he try an experimental drug for his illness. He agreed to the trial, and got better. I remember feeling so relieved that he was going to live.

Another stressful situation developed after he started to feel better. Melissa wanted to marry the man she was dating. This upset him terribly. He was jealous of another man spending time with his daughter. This was very difficult for me to understand and process. I felt Danny didn't like the fact that he could no longer control

Melissa. He had told her she couldn't date for a very long time. He wanted her to solely focus on raising their daughter and going to school. I encouraged him to allow Melissa to be happy, and that another man being in his daughter's life was inevitable. Danny always told me I didn't understand.

One afternoon Danny went to visit his daughter. He was not gone that long before he came home, and was very upset. I was concerned because he looked angry and as if he had been crying. He finally disclosed why he was so hurt. Apparently he had gone into the house and saw a framed picture of Melissa, Ann and Melissa's boyfriend, Steven. Danny said Steven was not part of his daughter's family, and displaying a picture of the three of them was very wrong. He said he pushed Melissa away when she tried to stop him from grabbing the picture. She ultimately threw him out of her house. He later told me she obtained a restraining order against him so he could no longer go to the house. I am uncertain if that was true.

I became infuriated after he told me why he was upset. I also could not believe how selfish and juvenile he was being at the time. Feeling awkward about another man being in your daughter's life was understandable. Being physically aggressive towards Melissa and throwing a fit about it, in front of his child nonetheless, was disgusting and unacceptable behavior. Danny was angry that I didn't support his actions. He said I didn't understand, and it was ultimately none of my business anyway. He left after I told him how I felt.

He returned home the following evening and proceeded to yell at me. He accused me of being an added stress he did not need. He stated I made no attempt to understand his pain, and was unsupportive. We had a physical altercation that evening. Danny kept pushing me around the apartment as he yelled at me. Every time I moved, he moved towards me. I was frightened, and had never seen him so angry, and full of rage. I pleaded with him to stop, and then begin to kick him away in my defense. I ran out of the apartment once he hit my face. It was the first time he had ever hit me in anger. At the time, I didn't consider how he kicked me at the house party during our first year together.

I drove all over town that night, and didn't know what to do. I was hurt, angry, and confused whether or not I was wrong for feeling the way I did. As it was, I had learned not to trust my own feelings. Finally, I went to my parent's house. My mother was up late, working in her office. I didn't tell her about the physical fight; however, I did ask if I could move back home. I explained that we were no longer getting along and the wedding was off. I could tell by the look on her face that she really didn't want me to come home. She was supportive anyway, and said   I could. I was humiliated that I had not planned better, and was unable to afford a place of my own.

I wish I could say that from that day on I stayed away from Danny. I believe my choice to move away again set the stage for meeting my current husband; however, it was a long 13 years before finding such a wonderful man.

Four

I lived with my parents for about six months before deciding to leave my hometown altogether. Danny had convinced me after the fight that I drove him to his rage because of my lack of understanding of his unique situation. He said he couldn't cope with how Melissa treated him, and fighting with me at the same time. He asked me to be more sensitive to his feelings so he wouldn't become angry. He never apologized for hurting me. Things calmed down between us, and we started dating again. This was our cycle of abuse. Things became heated; he blew up in one way or another, and then calmed down to gain my trust again. He felt he needed to be nice to me for a while in order to keep me in his life. He was no stranger to manipulation.

He was staying with his mother in the next town at that time. His step-father, Brad was a cardiologist, and wanted to purchase his own practice up north in

Sacramento. We both looked at this as an opportunity to start a new life in a bigger city, which offered more occupational opportunities. Danny moved in with his parents, and I moved in with my aunt in Sacramento.

I got a job working for a local hospital as a referrals coordinator for an out- patient children's clinic. Danny was not working, and felt he needed more time to recover from Valley Fever. Yet, he went fishing all the time, and seemed fine. I suppose he didn't have much motivation to work since his mother was supporting him, When he did work he bounced around from different positions. He tried working as an apprentice to an electrician, but was laid off after a few months. He started truck driving again, and had 10 different jobs over a 10 year period. Many laid him off, or he was hurt on the job, and spent some time on disability. That is still his pattern today at age 43.

I went home to visit my parents every chance I had; sometimes three weekends a month. Danny traveled with me half the time. I usually left Friday after work so I could stay with my parents for two nights. One time Danny went with me, and wanted us to stay the night in a hotel on the way. I didn't want to, and was anxious to visit with my family for as long as I could. I felt we could do that any other time. Danny kept pressing the issue. Finally, I said, "You may not have a good relationship with your parents, but I do. I want to see my family and spend time with them." That statement triggered a huge blow up. Danny was furious, and yelled at me. He called me every vulgar name there was, and said I was so wrong for saying that. I was frightened of him at that point. My whole body was trembling. I didn't know how to respond. I kept driving, and it was silent between us until we made it to my parent's house. A couple of days later he proceeded to make comments about the incident, and I felt guilty about my remark. I didn't say it to hurt him. I tried to convey the truth, and point out why it was so difficult for him to understand my relationship with my parents. I also think one of the reasons I went back home so often was because I hated my living situation in Sacramento.

Living with my aunt was difficult. Her house was located in a very bad neighborhood, and she went through my things while I was at work. My privacy was violated, and I never felt safe while I lived there. I rented an apartment after nine months of living with her. I was 25 years old, and that was the first time I did something on my own, without the help of my parents. Danny wasn't working at the time. He was able to help out with part of the rent, and I covered everything else.

The apartment I rented was small, but we loved it. It was located in a wooded area, and had a very peaceful atmosphere. We were happy at that time. We spent our time doing things we liked to do. We went fishing, bike riding, and to the movies. After about a year we decided to get married.

Many people told us we might as well get married since we had been together for seven years at that point. I never liked the idea of living together without being married. I was raised to believe it was wrong. Being a wife sounded appealing to me, and I thought I was in love. I felt we had been through so much together and mistook that for being a strong couple. I did not realize at the time that I simply tolerated Danny. I never should have gotten married, nor continued the relationship after the first couple of months.

Danny and I never had those crucial discussions couples need to have before living together or getting married. We never discussed our roles. Now I have realized he lacked the capacity to consider my feelings in the matter. He did, however, disclose early on how he felt women should do things to take care of their men. He claimed the Bible even spoke about a woman not being equal to a man, and should do as he desired. Danny never went to church, but attempted to quote the Bible if it was to his advantage. He informed me of how it would be a challenge for me when I became a mother. He said he expected me to take care of our child while making sure he never felt left out. He often made those kinds of statements which projected a great deal of selfishness.

Housework was always my responsibility as well. He refused to help me. I had a huge weight on my shoulders and did not realize it. I made the mistake of never asking myself what I wanted in a partner. I never thought about what kind of qualities I wanted in a man in order to have a fulfilling relationship. I accepted Danny for who he was and how he acted. I was not happy with much of his character, yet held on to him. I still struggle with why I was so drawn to him. I felt sorry for him a lot of the time, especially when he cried about how hurt he was over his childhood and his failures as an adult. I did not want to judge him. It was very confusing to see a person so down on themselves one minute, yet think they are intellectually

superior to the rest of the world the next.

Five

Danny was working again when we started planning our wedding. He was gone during the week, and travelled back and forth to Los Angeles. Our hometown was close to L.A. so he often spent time there visiting his best friend, Raymond. At the time Raymond was hanging out with a new group of women. Danny got close to them as well. He often stayed away when he could have come home so he could hang out over there. He told me what good people they were. Raymond was dating a girl named Stacy. She often spent time with three of her female friends who all lived together. Danny often joined them. I was very jealous again. I mentioned to him how I wish he would come home when he could so we could continue planning the wedding, and see each other. He had a way of turning things around, and blamed me for being selfish. A couple of times he said it was my behavior that kept him away. He said he didn't want to come home to a jealous woman. He claimed   there was nothing going on, and I should allow him to have friends. I felt like I was trying to smother him after we spoke about it. I never wanted to intervene with any of his friendships. I felt guilty about mentioning it. He usually had a way to devalue my needs.

Narcissists get bored very easily. We had been together for seven years at that point. It was time for him to look for attention elsewhere again. He was getting it from the women Raymond was around. This was the third time in our relationship that I knew of, he sought attention elsewhere. Danny often spoke of some of the struggles these women had and how he wanted to be there for them emotionally. He probably identified with them when it came to common problems. I was very confused. I tried to be supportive of his friendships, but it bothered me that he always took other people's feelings into consideration over mine.

Nonetheless, I continued to plan our wedding, and Danny told me how excited he was about it. I can't recall how I found out about it, but the public has the option of getting married on the grounds of the state capital. We both liked the idea, and reserved a spot. Danny's mother helped me find an Italian restaurant located in Old Town Sacramento for the reception. She went with me to taste the food. Everyone helped with the preparations for the event. Danny's aunts were very crafty, and made our wedding favors, the basket to hold the favors and ultimately decorated the area outside of the restaurant for the reception. My mother brought the table centerpieces. My dad hired mariachis to play at the reception. Danny's step-father did photography as a hobby and took all of our pictures that day. Danny's daughter was in our wedding as the flower girl. I felt a lot of love from both sides of the family. I had a horse and carriage take me and my wedding party to the capital. Both my parents walked me down the aisle, and both my sisters were bride's maids. It was a good day.

Danny did not put forth any money towards the wedding. Both of our parents helped and I saved a great deal for it. I often asked him to pitch in where he could, but he usually told me he didn't have enough. He did, however, want to pay for his two best men's tuxedos. He said he felt guilty making them pay for it because they had to travel out of town for our wedding. Raymond was one of the best men. He brought his girlfriend, Stacy. Stacy was a very nice woman and I liked her a lot.

Danny spent the night in the same hotel room as Raymond and Stacy the night before our wedding. At the wedding reception he told me how badly he felt for Stacy. He said she was crying that morning because Raymond did not want to marry her. Danny expressed a great deal of concern for her and brought it up throughout the reception. Danny also told me he wanted to hang out with all of his friends at the reception, and didn't want to feel obligated to only be with me. Although the day was great, that comment was one of the things that really bothered me. The other thing was Danny never told me that I looked good on our wedding day. I had to ask him what he thought. He said I looked fine. Compliments were not a part of his character, as it took attention away from him.

Danny cared very little for me. All the signs were there of someone whose sole focus was looking out for what he wanted. It has been difficult to digest; however, it's not because I am heartbroken. I am disappointed I wasted so much of my life, and tolerated someone who never deserved me. Nonetheless, I have learned that self- blame and dwelling are pointless.

Six

There are two areas in my life where I deeply regret my behavior. The first took place shortly after we were married. Danny nagged me about bringing another woman into our bed since the first couple of years we were together. He often brought it up, but dropped the issue for a while each time I expressed my disapproval. I didn't like the idea, and it made me feel as if I wasn't enough for him. I often felt like he had this great need for someone else. This wasn't because of my self-esteem; it's what he showed me. He stated it would be fun to experience together, and it would keep things interesting between us if we experimented a little. I always struggled with jealousy as it was, so I told him the only way I would entertain the thought was if we added another man into the picture as well. I didn't think he would go for it, but he did.

I felt Danny would continue to have interest in me if I were a little more open- minded, and willing to try new things. He said he did not want our marriage to go stale. This was just another way he manipulated me into doing what he wanted. We had only been married two months before we had sex with another couple.

We got involved with one of my friends who I worked with at the time. She often flirted with me at work, and she was married. I figured she was the best option. We started out by going to dinner with them to see how they acted outside the workplace. They were several years younger than we were, and fun to be around. They invited us to their home where they had a jacuzzi.

They asked us to join them, and said no one was allowed to wear swimsuits. The details are irrelevant; however, that was the night I started my polyamorous lifestyle. I was intimate with both of them, as Danny only had sex with women.

We messed around with those two for a couple of months. They came to our house, and often had us over to spend the night. We actually developed a nice friendship. But, the couple started to show more interest in me, and Danny became pushy with them. He asked to go over all the time. If we saw them in the mall together, he decided it as an opportunity to invite himself to their home. The couple grew tired of him, because he seemed clingy. The one downfall about hanging out with those two was they fought quite a bit, even in public. I used that as a reason to stop doing what we were doing with them, and to move on with our lives. Danny agreed as I knew he felt the growing tension they had towards him.

I felt it was an experience we got out of our system and could move on. Danny didn't want to stop that lifestyle. On line he found a group of people who did that sort of thing. They got together once a month for a dance in a banquet room at a Howard Johnson Hotel. Danny signed us up to be members, and we went to a dance. He felt it was my responsibility to seek out the other couple, and said it was too intimidating if the male was the aggressor. The truth was, he was too much of a coward to put himself out there, and wanted me to take all the risks. I felt like I was single again, and did not want to do it. He told me to stop being boring, and to dance with other women. He wanted me to pick out who we could possibly start to "date." I was the one who had to risk rejection and humiliation while he sat there and watched me from the table. It was humiliating putting myself out there, asking women to dance, and flirting with them. That was not what I wanted for my life. But then, something happened.

I received a lot of attention, and started to develop many friends. Most of the couples met there to potentially hook up for the night; however, there were also couples who wanted to be intimate, and have a friendship as well. It felt great to be around people who were not putting me down, or negative towards me. I felt if I had to be in that lifestyle, I was going to enjoy it any way I was able. I tried to develop a connection. We became really close with one couple in particular. Their names were Ryan and Carrie. They not only wanted to sleep with us, they wanted us in their lives. I was more attracted to Carrie, and became quite fond of her.

This all lasted for about three months. We went out and met different couples, even though we often stayed the night with Ryan and Carrie. There was another couple we were intimate with, but they both became too emotionally attached to us. I grew uncomfortable about it, and we stopped seeing them. That was a very different lifestyle than I had ever experienced. Many problems can develop when crossing boundaries with other people's spouses. There was jealousy, misunderstandings, and secrets. At one point Danny said it would be ok if the two of us had sex with other people in separate rooms from each other. That hurt me because it was then when I realized the sexual play no longer had anything to do with us as a couple.

I also realized we were amongst people just like us. They were not completely happy with their spouse, and used swinging as a means to safely seek out others. I was deeply troubled that my own husband did not have a problem watching me have sex with another man and woman. I do take ownership for my part in all of that. I was not forced into it. Originally, I agreed to it to get along in my marriage. Then I ended up enjoying it- mainly the comforting relationship I gained out of it. I did enjoy the sexual aspect of it as well.

I was 27 years old, and it was during that time in my life when I decided I did not want to have children. I enjoyed going out and doing things on the weekends, and didn't want to be a mother. Deep down I felt the experience of motherhood would not have been a pleasant one while married to Danny.

Seven

I elected to have a tubal ligation. My gynecologist stated he was not comfortable doing the procedure on a young, attractive, and healthy woman. So he asked my husband to come into the office so he could ask what he thought of my decision. I didn't agree with that protocol because it was my body. Danny said he felt badly for me because I would never know the feeling of becoming a mother. Nonetheless, he supported the decision so it was not an issue. My doctor also wanted me to get approval from my primary care doctor. He stated he wanted another doctor to approve it and support this decision. He was also concerned I may regret the procedure later on in life. I went to see my primary care doctor. He asked me if I had experienced any psychological trauma that would impact my decision not to have children. I said no, and he was fine with it. It was that easy. He called my other doctor from the exam room and gave his approval.

I was able to schedule the procedure for a couple of weeks out. Part of the protocol is to take a pregnancy test. I took one and it was negative. We were supposed to abstain from intercourse until the procedure; however, Danny wouldn't leave me alone. He had needs. They offered me another pregnancy test the day of the procedure, which I declined. My periods were always irregular, and I was told I only ovulated a few times a year. I felt a pregnancy test at that point was redundant.

I had the procedure, and the following week felt nauseated all the time. My breasts started to hurt, and I became extremely emotional. My parents came for a weekend visit, and I cried when they left. That was completely out of character for me. I was also exhausted throughout the day. I called my doctor and told him how sick I felt. He told me not to worry, and stated that sometimes the anesthesia from the procedure can make you sick. It wasn't the effects from the anesthesia; I was pregnant.

We found out Christmas Eve morning when I took an in-home pregnancy test. Initially I was not excited about it. I immediately said that I was not going to have the baby, and would get an abortion. (My first reaction was something Danny made sure my daughter knew of since a very young age). I felt having a child was out of the question. I spoke out of fear. Danny was very excited and pleaded with me to reconsider. We went to his mother's house to visit, and I slept on and off throughout the day as I was exhausted. Everyone kept asking me what was wrong, and I stated I was just tired. We didn't say anything to anyone about the pregnancy. Danny kept asking me to change my mind when I was awake. He said this baby was meant to be.

I changed my mind by the time we returned home that evening. This was not by his influence. The initial

shock had worn off, and I realized there was a baby inside of me. It was my baby. Everyone in the family knew I had the procedure not to have children. So, they were all quite surprised about our news. I called my mother that night, and she cried. She was very happy for me.

I received mixed reactions of my pregnancy news from people at work. The doctors I worked for were surprised and confused since they knew I took some time off for my tubal ligation. There were also some women who were unsuccessfully trying to get pregnant. They were not pleased with me since I took measures not to have children, and then ended up pregnant.

I enjoyed every moment of my pregnancy, and read as much information as I could. I learned about what was going on inside my body, and my baby's development. I knew it was going to be the only time in my life I would experience this miracle. So, I appreciated being blessed with it. Danny came with me to my first few doctors' appointments to see an ultrasound of the baby. We both had fun buying items, and preparing for our daughter. We found out the sex because I wanted to plan. I did not name my daughter; my mother-in-law thought of the name and pressed for our acceptance. Danny insisted our daughter's middle name be his name, but with an "a" at the end. We named her Chloe.

For the most part Danny was good to me while I was pregnant. He was in love with the idea of having a baby. We were really excited to meet her, and agreed on several issues when it came to raising our child. Neither one of us cared for a few ways our parents were with us. So, we promised each other to be different with Chloe. We planned to never talk baby talk to her, and always treat her like a little person. I believe this helped develop her vocabulary and her conversation skills at a young age. I think Danny felt this was an opportunity to make up for his failures with his first daughter. He used the fights he had with Melissa as a reason not to see Ann a great deal of the time. He blamed her, and stated she made it too difficult to see her. Unfortunately, missing out on a lot of Ann's life was one more behavior of which he never took ownership. Ann grew up much closer to her step-father.

My pregnancy was uneventful and healthy. Chloe was a large baby, so I had to maneuver in a wheelchair at work during the last couple of months, as I was in a great deal of pain. That part was the only complaint I had about my pregnancy.

Between my mother and two different groups of women at work I had three baby showers. We had a lot of help and support, and it was much appreciated. That was probably the only time Danny did not act is if it was owed to him. He expressed his appreciation as well.

My last doctor's visit was about three weeks before I was due. He told me the baby would be nine pounds at birth if I waited the full 40 weeks. He suggested inducing labor two weeks early. I liked the idea of an elective procedure instead of unexpectedly going into labor in the middle of the night. The following week I checked into the hospital about eight in the morning. My mother and mother-in-law were there with us throughout the day. Chloe would not budge, so they had to give me the injection to induce my labor twice. We kicked our parents out when it was time to push. We wanted the moment she came into the world to be between us. Danny was very supportive during the birth. He told me several times how proud he was of me. It felt great to hear those words coming from him. He had never said anything like that to me before. I gave birth by 10PM that same day.

Chloe weighed eight pounds, 11 ounces. She was very alert, and looked all around the room within minutes of her birth. They put her in my arms and my whole world changed. I have never felt so much love for anyone or anything in my entire life. I felt so complete with my daughter in my arms.

I was unable to go on disability after having the baby. We couldn't afford the decrease in income. Luckily the group of doctors I worked for were very generous, and allowed me to do my job from home for two months. So, technically, I had three days off of work after having Chloe. I was relieved I had the opportunity to make money while at home on maternity leave. It was nice being able to bond with my baby as well. My mother stayed with us for a couple of weeks. She was a huge help, as she cooked several meals and froze them for us so I wouldn't have to cook. I had the majority of the responsibilities at home after she left. I worked in between feedings, cleaning, cooking and washing clothes. Danny went to work and came home and spent time with the baby. That frustrated me. His idea of helping me was holding Chloe so I could do everything else.

I felt so much joy in being a mother, and appreciated any time I had with my daughter. We were always taking pictures of her as well, so I started scrapbooking with them. I had never been the crafty type with much imagination for creating; however, I did quite well with this hobby, and enjoyed it. I also started writing a journal to my baby. I wanted to be able to share all the feelings I had about her growth, personality, and her activities when she got older.

Chloe was only four months old when Danny wanted to start seeing other couples again. I didn't want to, and was done with that way of life. I wanted to be home with my baby, and enjoy family time between the three of us. Danny would not let it go. He asked his mother to keep Chloe overnight while we went out. That hurt me, because I didn't want to be away from my baby; especially to go out with other couples. We went to another dance, and saw many of the couples we knew before I got pregnant. I danced while Danny sat at a table and drank. I was no longer interested in being in that kind of environment. I went through the motions of talking to people and was friendly, but I had no intention of doing anything that night. I eventually told Danny I was really tired and wanted to go home. That made him angry. He argued with me to stay and try to "hook up." I was persistent and told him I wanted to go home. We went home, and he pouted. He didn't speak to me the rest of the night. In the morning he blamed his behavior on the alcohol. That was the last dance we ever attended.

Danny was badly injured on the job some time before Chloe turned a year old. He was seated in a forklift which was attached to the back of a flatbed trailer. The forklift was about three or four feet off the ground. Somehow he managed to eject the forklift from the trailer, and it fell straight to the ground with him seated in it. The impact damaged several of his lower vertebrae. I do not have any proof, but I often wondered if he did this on purpose. He hated working there, or working at all. I felt he looked for a way out. The individuals who worked there tried making that same scenario happen again after his accident. No one could figure out how the forklift ejected. Needless to say, that ended his employment for several years. The one advantage was he was able to stay home with Chloe, and she did not have to go into daycare for a while.

Danny often sent me pictures of Chloe during the day while I was at work. He kept me well informed of what she was doing. I missed her a great deal. It was comforting to know she was with one of us. Coming home after work was difficult because there was more work to do. Danny only took care of Chloe and played with her. He refused to do laundry, cook or clean. That was my job.

I wanted to leave Danny by the time my daughter was two years old. It was then when I recognized how selfish he was. I was very confused about my feelings towards him. I thought I loved him, but was disgusted with him at the same time. He was being paid by workman's compensation or disability; I lost track. He spent his extra money on a hobby. He liked racing remote control cars at a little speedway close to where we lived. That was not a cheap hobby. The cars, remote control and upkeep were very expensive. One night he came home after being at the mini track, and looked incredibly guilty. I asked him what was wrong. He told me the battery in his little car died in the middle of a race. They had parts there at the store inside the raceway. He bought a battery on the spot to replace it. It was over $50. He said he felt terrible about making the purchase. He was depressed about it for the rest of the night, but did nothing to change his spending habits going forward. Danny never gave me money for diapers or anything my daughter needed. Worrying about that was my department.

One of the many difficult aspects of parenting a child with someone who is narcissistic is the feeling of being a single parent. I could not count on him for anything. I wanted to expose Chloe to as much of the world as I could. I wanted to take her to the zoo and do all the fun things parents do with their children. Danny went with us to the zoo once. He refused to go with us after the initial experience, and stated there was no reason for him to go since the zoo didn't offer him any entertainment. He was only focused on was how he could benefit from experiences. Watching his daughter enjoy herself was not something he saw as a benefit.

We did enjoy some nice family moments. One day we went on a day trip to Reno. We drove around all day. Chloe was almost three years old at the time. She handled the car ride very well, and was delightful. We stopped and took a kayak ride on the lake. I was very hesitant because of my fear of water. I cannot   swim. Danny pushed for me to go anyway. I was up front, Chloe was in the middle, and Danny was in the rear. Chloe loved it and reached over to put her hand in the water. I tolerated it because she was having such a great time. We were on the water for a half an hour when I said I had enough. Danny mentioned he was glad I tolerated the ride, and we were able to experience the ride as a family. Moments like that helped me believe we could continue to be happy. It was one of the reasons I wouldn't give up.

There was a year-long period when Chloe was three or four when she was sick all of the time. Sometimes Danny was working, and other times he was in between jobs. I was always the one who had to stay home with Chloe if she was sick, even if Danny was home. He claimed she needed me more. I didn't have any support from him. I am the one who took her to different doctors to try to find out what was wrong with her. She had flu-like symptoms, and lacked a great deal of energy. Chloe was in daycare at the time, so the doctors told me the sickness was because she was around other children. I knew that wasn't the case. I was terribly worried about her, to the point it physically affected me. I had chest pains a lot due to the stress of not knowing how to help her. I felt alone in the matter.

Chloe became sick one weekend when we were out of town, and visiting my parents for Christmas. Christmas Eve she had a high fever, and was complaining her ear hurt. Danny told me Chloe wasn't that bad off, and we shouldn't go to the emergency room like I suggested. We went after a great deal of arguing. That was a nightmare, because half the town was there as well. The stress was unbelievable between worrying about Chloe enduring so much pain, and dealing with Danny's complaints about spending Christmas Eve in the E.R. I had two children!

We ultimately found out what was causing Chloe's perpetual illness. Her primary care doctor ordered a CT scan of her sinuses, and found her adenoids to be too large. They were not allowing her sinuses to drain, so she was always sick with a fever, ear infection, sore throat, and a runny nose. We took her for an adenoidectomy, and it resolved the problem.

I could go on forever about the different scenarios which played out in regards to my lack of support and selfish behavior from my ex-husband; however I believe I have made my point.

Eight

When Chloe was very young Danny and I "purchased" a large house with his mother and step-father. My parents gave me several thousand dollars for our part in the down payment. The agreement was we would all live there for a few years, and then sell it. Then Danny and I could afford to get our own home from the profit we made off the house. The plan did not go as we expected. Our names were not on the loan, nor the deed of the house. This was something my in-law both dismissed. We were also supposed to get a tax break, as homeowners are allowed. My father-in-law stated he would give us money at the end of every year to make up for it. That also never happened. That decision was one of the worst mistakes I have ever made. I hated living with them. The house was a model home in a wealthy part of town. My mother- in-law told me she felt rich. The house was beautiful, and a bit over the top. It had all the upgrades as well. I am not materialistic by any means. I grew to hate the house and what it stood for.

We "looked" like we were rich. That was not of any importance to me. We had our own living quarters, which were much smaller than what Danny's parents had. We shared the kitchen, but his mother took over all of the decorating. They also made all the decisions regarding the house. I felt like a child living with my parents. The only thing I liked was Chloe had her own room, and it was large.

About six months after moving in, I realized I had little control over most aspects of my life. Danny undermined me as a parent in front of Chloe, and the house I lived in wasn't mine. I didn't have any respect for my husband, and felt trapped. I had planned on staying in the marriage until Chloe was 18 years old. I felt I owed it to her, and didn't want to disrupt her life.

Another part of my struggle was because we lived in a house which my parents had a lot of money invested. How could I leave? I also lacked the confidence in myself to live on my own. I didn't realize I had always been alone, and handled everything independently. I also didn't realize that I made enough money to support myself and my daughter. My self-esteem was extremely crippled; I didn't see how I could manage on my own.

There were many nights when I prayed to God to take my life. I felt so hopeless, and didn't want to wake up most mornings. I didn't know how I was going to survive, and keep my sanity. I gained a lot of weight, and was miserable. I was so tired of my husband's negativity about everything, and the way he treated me.

I started going to school again the last couple of years we were together. I worked all day, and went to school one night a week. I got home after 10PM on school nights, and still had to take care of household responsibilities. My mother-in- law helped me a great deal with Chloe. She often picked her up from after-school care and fed her dinner for me. Danny always had something else to do, like sit on the couch, play on-line poker, or watch television. His mother often complained to me that he was a loser. I later found out she mentioned something to Danny when I was down stairs doing laundry on a school night. She expressed her disapproval of his laziness, and told him I shouldn't be doing laundry after working all day and going to school. He told her to mind her own business.

One evening my mother-in-law and I were in the kitchen and she brought up something her sister mentioned to her. They were discussing how I was going to school to ultimately obtain my Master's degree, and Danny was always going to be undereducated. They spoke about how it would be difficult for me because of the incongruence of our intellect. My mother-in- law asked how I was going to handle that. I told her it was already something I had been struggling with for years. You couldn't have a meaningful conversation with Danny. He was right, and you were wrong if you expressed a difference in opinion. Danny used to criticize me for speaking the way I did. He said, "No one talks like that. You sound stupid. Why can't you use simple words like everyone else?" He was essentially asking me to dumb myself down when speaking to him. Yet, he did so in a way to put me down. At the time I didn't know what a narcissist was. I just knew he was a jerk.

Nine

Danny found truck driving to increasingly hurt his back. So, he decided to try something new, and applied for a job as a poker dealer. He was hired by a casino about 45 minutes away from where we lived. I didn't care for the profession, because his income was dependent upon how much he was tipped by the players. Nonetheless, I was supportive, because he really liked it. It was the first time he was employed somewhere, and didn't complain about it. He also said he was happy there because the environment provoked him to be social. He felt more outgoing, confident, and enjoyed making people laugh.

He was making a good amount of money for the first time in his life. He even started to exhibit more confidence on a daily basis. We planned to take a cruise about five months after he started working at the casino. Each week we saved more and more money for the trip. This was also the first time Danny ever saved for something. My in-laws took care of Chloe so we could have a vacation as a couple. We were both excited because we had never taken a cruise.

Things felt awkward between us when we arrived on the ship. I couldn't identify what it was at the time. We walked all over as the ship left the dock. I wanted to have sex as soon as we arrived in our room. Again, it was very awkward. He seemed to be in unfamiliar territory. The encounter felt forced, and was unsatisfying. I was frustrated, so I asked him what was wrong. He said there was nothing wrong, and dismissed my concerns.

It was a three-night cruise to Ensenada, Mexico. There was gambling on the ship, and Danny often planted himself at a poker table. I was alone a lot of the time the ship was moving. I tried to stay positive, as he did what he wanted. I went shopping and went to comedy shows by myself. We did have fun when we docked in Mexico. We saw the Blowhole in La Bufadora, walked around all day, and shopped. I enjoyed the vacation besides the odd feelings between us. Danny appeared to as well.

Our relationship significantly declined after the cruise. He wasn't affectionate with me at all anymore. We stopped having sex, and he often stayed the night in the same town where the casino was located. He told me he was tired of driving back and forth, and one of the male poker dealers let him stay at his place. His name was Tom. He started hanging out at the casino on his days off, and said he and several workers liked to go bowling over there as well. I asked if he would take me along with him so we could spend time together. He told me I wouldn't fit in with the crowd as they were mostly younger Asian men and women. According to him, I didn't fit in with anyone. The last time I checked, he wasn't Asian either.

I asked Danny several times if he was having an affair. He denied it, and even made jokes about it. I checked our cell phone bill, and noticed there was a number on there he was spending a lot of time calling and texting. A female answered when I called the number. I hung up, and approached him about it. Danny exploded and cussed me out. He claimed it was Tom's number, and that was probably his girlfriend who answered. He said he was disgusted in me for not trusting him. I was so confused and felt horrible for checking up on him. I didn't know what to do. All the signs were there, but I couldn't prove it. Do you leave a marriage because of assumptions you are making? I didn't take into consideration that he had made my life hell even before that incident. I think I needed proof for myself to finally leave him.

One evening Chloe and I met him for dinner before he had to leave for work. His shift was from midnight to eight in the morning. We ate at Red Robin. He and I used to try to take the honey mustard sauce from each other because we each liked it so much. That evening I reached over to act like I was going to grab his sauce. I was attempting to be playful, but accidently spilled it on the table. As a result, he kicked me several times. He was furious, and told me I was stupid. So many emotions ran through my body. I was angry, hurt and frightened of the hateful monster I had married. Chloe was six years old at the time. She was busy coloring, and did not pay attention to what happened. I tried my best not to cry and remained calm. I packed her up and we left as soon as she was done eating.

It was a couple of months later when I went to Disneyland with Chloe and my sister, Elizabeth. Danny was working or gone a great deal of the time, and I wanted to take Chloe to have some fun. We went a couple of days after Christmas. We had a really nice time and it was a much needed trip. We were in the car with my sister, heading back to where she lived when Danny called me. He was crying, and said he had gotten fired from the casino. He was very upset and unclear about what happened. I remember thinking, "now what are we going to do?" I told him we would discuss it when I got back home. I was very embarrassed that my sister had to hear the conversation but, it couldn't be helped. She didn't show any judgment, and was very supportive about it.

I arrived home the following day. Danny told me he got into an argument with a female employee in the break room a couple of weeks prior. He said she had approached him about a rumor going around the casino about her that he had started. Supposedly, she was angry with him, confronted him, and walked off. Danny said he tried to stop her to tell her it wasn't true. He said he tried to touch her shoulder, and missed, thus grabbing her long hair. There are cameras everywhere in the casino, even in the break rooms. He said management looked at that as an assault, and said they would see if they were going to take action against him. He hadn't told me any of that until they made their decision to fire him. I didn't question the story he told me. I was stressed out about the fact that we had bills to pay, a daughter to take care of, and now he was out of work.

A few days later the casino informed us they were going to deny unemployment payments due to the nature of his termination. They also banned him from the casino as a customer for 30 days. Danny claimed that was ridiculous, and they were being unfair to him. The only way they would reconsider was if the victim wrote a letter stating it was not an assault. I asked Danny if he knew how to get a hold of her. He said he would be able to find her because he knew her brother. I told him to go take care of it, and he left to the town where the casino was located. He ended up spending the night, and claimed to stay with Tom.

The following day he brought a letter home, and asked me to fax it to the unemployment office along with the appeal paperwork. The woman had typed the letter stating they were just having a discussion, and he did not harm her. She also signed her name, and left her telephone number at the bottom. It was the same number I found on our phone bill, and called several months prior. I felt sick to my stomach. It was such an unreal moment. Finally, everything came crashing down. Here was my proof, and I was devastated. He got fired for fighting at work with his lover.

I approached him about it, and he said she was just a friend. He said they had gotten close, but he hadn't had an affair with her. I didn't believe him because of his behavior over the past several months. Danny didn't give it a second thought. He told me there was nothing going on and to drop it. I was miserable and felt betrayed. I was a good wife, and always supported him, despite what he lacked in a partner. I didn't deserve to feel that way.

We argued a lot over the next several weeks. I cried to him about his betrayal, and how much it hurt me. One evening we were sitting in the living room, and he was listening to me, but admitting nothing. He sighed and said he was growing tired of listening to my little "poor- me sessions." I don't know why I expected anything different from him, but it still crushed me.

Danny finally got paid from the unemployment office and decided to get a tattoo of a dragon on his chest. Not that catching up on bills would be a priority. After he got the tattoo he said he wanted to go show his friend, Tom. He said he hadn't seen him since he was fired, and knew he would appreciate the visit. I didn't catch it at the time, but it was Tom who he supposedly spent the night with when he went and got the letter. Danny returned from Tom's house a few hours later, and looked distraught. He wouldn't tell me what was wrong, and kept to himself. He was outside on the phone for the rest of the night. I was inside the house with Chloe, trying to hold back tears. I had no idea what was happening.

The following morning I got to work, and one of my closest girlfriends, Janelle, wanted to talk to me. She appeared very nervous, and said we needed to take a walk together. She was struggling a bit with if she should tell me the news. On our walk she told me Danny had called her the night before and told her everything that was going on. Janelle was my friend I met at work when Chloe was first born. Danny was not that close to her. She was just as shocked as I was that he reached out to her. She was unaware he did not have anyone else. She told me he admitted to her he had been having an affair with a Cambodian woman named, Rim who worked at the casino. He said she had persistently asked him to leave me over the last couple of months. Danny told her he wouldn't leave me, and he didn't want to be a step-father to her two children. Apparently she started messing around with another poker dealer to make Danny jealous, and that was what their fight was about that was caught on tape. He was upset when he got home from Tom's house, because he saw Rim's car parked outside. Apparently, she had decided to mess around with him as well. He was heartbroken, and called my friend to discuss his pain.

The story seems so unreal now that I have typed out the entire scenario; however, this is how everything came unfolded. Danny never considered the humiliation and pain he put me through; nor did he consider how inappropriate it was to call my friend to cry about the woman with whom he cheated. The fact that he had a family which he tore apart was never mentioned.

I was very upset, and had to leave work. I called Danny on my way home and asked if he was in our bedroom. He said he was. I told him I knew everything, to start packing his stuff, and to get the hell out of the house. I said I was on my way home. He said, "Good, then you can watch me kill myself."

Ten

March 13, 2008 was the day I came home early from work to end my marriage. I went upstairs, and Danny was sitting on the couch. I sat on the chair by the desk, about six feet away from him. I told him, "I don't want to be married to you anymore." He said, "Then I'm going to kill myself, and you are going to help." He rose from the couch and had a knife in his hand. I tried to run downstairs to get away from him, but he grabbed me by the arm, threw me on the couch, and sat on me. He said, "You are going to stab me." He grabbed one of my hands and placed it on the knife, which was pointing at his stomach. I was terrified. I wouldn't have a problem with him dying; however, it was not going to be by my hands. I struggled to get him off of me. He weighed over 200 pounds, so it was very difficult. I managed to inch my way out from under him, and practically flew downstairs. I didn't care if I fell. My focus was to get from our living room, to the bottom of the stairs, so I could run out the front door. I made it to the family room downstairs when he caught up with me, and grabbed my hair. He dragged me up the stairs, holding on to my hair. I was terrified and in a great deal of pain. I remember thinking it was so unreal that all of it was happening. He threw my car keys on top of the entertainment center so I couldn't reach them. He tried to trap me any way he could. The fight between us lasted for two hours. It consisted of the same scenario I just described, over and over. He aggressively pushed me to the ground, the couch or against the wall while squeezing my arms. He treated me like a rag doll.

Finally, I realized I needed to do something differently, or I was going to die. I told him I gave up. I said, "Maybe it doesn't have to be over, and we can find a way to work this out." He fell for it, and immediately stopped fighting me. I was not sure what was more terrifying, the attack, or the fact he was so demented, and believed me. We talked for a little bit, and he discussed his pain over his ex-girlfriend's betrayal. He compared her to a cockroach that needed to be sprayed with Raid. He had just beaten me up, and he was having a pity party. He never apologized for hurting me that day, or any day. A few weeks later I pointed out his abusive behavior. He said it was my fault because I tried to get away.

I was in a complete fog, and was not sure what I was going to do. I didn't have any money saved, as we always struggled financially. I went and picked up my daughter from school and continued life as usual. I went to work the following day covered with bruises all over my arms and legs. I hid them.

That evening I was taking a shower when I noticed a black line on the right side of me. At first I thought it was my long hair in the way, but it wouldn't go away. I got out of the shower, and continued to see it. Something was on my eye. It seemed as though my vision had changed as well. I became very nervous, because I thought I was having a stroke. Danny took me to the emergency room. He told me to lie if they asked about the bruises on my arms. He said to tell them I got into a fight with some women at work. I was seen, and my bruises were not discovered. The doctors told me I suffered from a retinal tear. They stated it could have been caused from grunting or trying to push against extreme pressure. It was from trying to get the 200 pound monster off of me for a couple of hours. I had to endure a couple of sessions of very painful laser treatments to correct the problem. Danny blamed me for that as well. He said, "If you hadn't tried to get away, it wouldn't have happened."

Eleven

The last seven months were very difficult, confusing and shameful. Danny moved to our old hometown to work as a poker dealer. He stayed with one of my sisters and her husband. I enjoyed the break from him; however, his absence negatively affected Chloe. She missed him and cried a lot. I received a phone call from a parent of one of her friends. She said Chloe cried in school when talking to her friends about missing her dad. Danny hadn't called her very often when he was away. I was very confused about leaving with Chloe, and hurting her even more. My heart sank whenever I thought about it. After a few months she was used to his absence, and her feelings towards him hardened. She stayed a couple of weeks with my parents during that time; so she was in the same town as he was. Danny didn't visit her. My mother told me she asked Chloe if she wanted to call her dad, but Chloe declined. I feel she was mad at him.

Meanwhile, I lost all the weight I had gained because of the depression. I started walking every day and lost 35 pounds. I applied for a medical credit card, and had plastic surgery to enlarge my breasts as well. I wanted to feel good about myself. Danny had torn me down for so long, and betrayed me. I needed something to help lift me up.

My sister threw Danny out after a few months. She realized he wasn't making any attempts to save money and get a place of his own. That humiliated me, and I didn't blame her. She opened up her home to help us out, and he took advantage of them by getting way too comfortable. So, he moved in with his cousin, James. He also started selling drugs. Methamphetamines were the drug of choice in our hometown. I did not approve of that at all, but knew he would do as he wanted, regardless.

Danny told me about a money opportunity James was considering. He heard about a website which   showed women flirting with the on-line users, and touching themselves. He said you had to pay if you wanted to see them take off their clothes and play with sex toys. He said James wanted to set up a camera in his house and have different women come in and work, and he would take a portion of the profit. He basically wanted to be an on-line pimp.

Danny suggested I get into it since I looked really good. He complimented me and said I looked very young for being 34 and I had a nice body. I liked the way I looked as well, and it was nice to finally get recognition from my spouse. I didn't see it as manipulation on his part. He wanted to make money off of me. My state of mind was very unhealthy at that point. I had been beaten down emotionally and physically, and was expected to move passed it without any resolution. I was also in a loveless marriage and felt trapped. What I did next was the second behavior I spoke of deeply regretting.

Danny wasn't making a lot of money at the casino, or at selling drugs, so he moved back home without a job. He purchased an expensive camera so he could put me on-line. We also went and bought several different lingerie outfits I could wear. He contacted this guy named, Blake, who helped us connect and work for the site. We had to download an application on our computer, and he gave me ideas on what kind of things to say to the customers. The most disturbing thing he stated was there were going to be child molesters watching in the chat rooms. Blake's said, "it's better they are in there watching you than hunting children."

Chloe had come home from my parents' house that week as well. One of the things she mentioned was that Danny was not a good dad. She said it one day while she was playing. Danny immediately took offense, and accused my parents of feeding her the thought. The same week I also received an email from my mother. She sent it to our joint email account not realizing we both read it. She stated her disgust in Danny's lack of attention to Chloe while he and she were in my mom's hometown. She mentioned how he took advantage of living with my sister, didn't treat me very well, or provided for our family. She said, "Something needs to change!" He and I both read the email at the same time. Danny took the laptop from me, and started writing back to my mother. He said he told her she would never see Chloe again.

I was furious that my mother put me in that situation. I did not disagree with a word she said. But, I was still married to him, living in the same house, and didn't know what to do. I felt I was powerless to make any changes. Danny never listened to me, or did anything at my request. I think what happened next was I went into survival mode. I was angry at my mom and didn't understand why. Danny threw a fit and said how stupid my parents were. I felt an amazing amount of pressure on me.

My mom called after she received the email. I started screaming at her. I told her she had no right to say what she did. My mother kept calling me crazy while on the phone. She kept saying, "You are acting crazy." It made it worse, because I was going crazy. I didn't look at this as a time to ask for help. As it was, I still was uncertain if I was actually abused. I didn't see it like that just yet. I told her I hated her and wanted her out of my life. Danny was right there, and smiling. I didn't realize what I was doing and was fueled by rage. My rage was misdirected at my mom. That was on my 35th birthday in July. I wrote one final email to my sisters and my parents after the call. I called everyone out on all of their messy lives, and told them all to go to hell. I was numb after that.

The following week I started performing on-line. I was really nervous the first time I logged on to my account to be watched by others. It was a lot easier than I anticipated. All I could see was a black screen. Then various user names started popping up, typing messages to get my attention. Most of them were complimenting me and telling me how hot I was. It's embarrassing to say, but I enjoyed it. I looked at it as positive attention. I was in private chat when all the user names disappeared and only one remained.

Sometimes the customer would allow me to see him as well. The customer told me what to do to myself, and I did it. I've always been a very sexual person, so I cannot say this was miserable for me. I didn't take into consideration how low I was sinking and degrading myself. My main goal was to make money so I could start a new life, and get out of my marriage. Danny later told me, because of his betrayal, he felt he owed it to me to allow attention from other guys.

My on-line job lasted about three months before I quit. It was too overwhelming with performing on the internet late at night, my day job, going to school and being a mother. I did make friends with three men from the site, and we talked often. I ended up having an emotional affair with one of them. He lived out of state, and gave me the emotional connection I desperately needed. He never asked me for anything, and wanted to be there for me. We developed a very nice friendship.

One day in August I was at work, and it just hit me; I was done. I had reached my limit, and was not going to live in hell for the rest of my life. I chuckled a bit, because I felt a huge weight lifted. I told my friend, Janelle, and she was really happy to hear my decision. She said I could do it, and she would be there to support me in any way she could. That day I started strategizing.

I needed Danny out of the house in order to plan my escape. I helped him find a truck driving job which took him far away. He was gone for more than a week at a time. That gave me time to think and plan. The problem was Danny grew very insecure about our relationship by that time. I had hastily told him it would be well deserved if I slipped and had an affair. He called me every half hour throughout the day. I tried acting like everything was ok when he did come home, but I had trouble knowing what normal was supposed to look like anymore. Danny continued having sex with me, and I wanted to vomit every time. I hated him and my life there in that house.

By September, with my tail in between my legs, I called and asked my mother for help. I told her all about the abuse, how I wanted to leave, but starting over was expensive. My mother was shocked about everything I told her. She said she knew things weren't right, but had no idea the abuse was to that degree. She told me how hurt she and my dad had been since throwing them out of my life. She also said she understood my frame of mind, and   deposited $5,000 in my checking account the following day. I withdrew it the same day, hoping Danny wouldn't find out. He questioned me when he saw the transaction on-line.   I told him the bank had made an error and called me, because I had to withdraw it and give it back. Thank God he believed me.

I was able to start planning once I had the funds. I told my in-laws I was leaving because I needed to purchase items and keep them in the garage. My father-in- law stated, "I'm surprised you stayed this long." They both knew their son was a complete ass. Everyone was willing to help me. I also told Danny's Aunt Carmen I was leaving him. I wanted to live on her side of town, so she helped me look for an apartment. Everyone I told understood why I wanted to leave. They had all seen how he treated me, and how good I was to him. I rented a post office box, purchased another cell phone, rented an apartment, and registered my daughter for another school.

My new life was scheduled to take place on November 1, 2008. That was the day I was able to move into my apartment, and Chloe would start school the following day. I filed for divorce on our ninth wedding anniversary, which was in the middle of October. I did so because I was given 30 days from filing to serve Danny with the paper work. I had planned on having him served after I left. I was going to leave when he was at work, and knew he would head home when he found out.

He left back to work the day after I filed for divorce. It was always difficult for him to leave Chloe. He often cried before he headed back on the road. I couldn't have cared less. That evening he and my mother- in-law were both in Chloe's bedroom as he was kissing her good night. He started crying again, and his mother hugged him. It took every ounce of my being to abstain from rolling my eyes, and calling him a little bitch. It angered me how he did that in front of Chloe. My daughter always worried about her dad, and wanted him to be ok. Their parent/child roles were reversed.

I had to drive Danny out to his diesel truck which was 30 minutes away. I was quiet during the entire drive. All I could think about was, it was the last time I was going to see that son of a bitch. We arrived at the truck, and I helped him off with his personal items. He started crying again and asked me, "What are you doing? What are you planning? Why are you being so cold?" I was irritated, and asked what he was talking about. He pointed out my distant behavior. I told him I wasn't acting any differently, and dismissed his concerns. Treating him that way felt extremely liberating. He looked very upset, got in the truck, and drove off. I felt ecstatic to be rid of him.

Twelve

I took Chloe out for dinner one evening the following week. I shut my phone off because I was tired of getting Danny's calls every 30 minutes. I wanted a nice uninterrupted visit with my daughter. I put my phone back on when we got home. I had 12 missed calls from Danny. He left me a rude message saying how fucked up I was for shutting off my phone. He called right after I listened to his message. He yelled at me, and asked what I was doing. I told him why I shut my phone off, and he didn't believe me. We went back and forth for a few minutes, and then I had enough. I told him to fuck off, broke my phone in half, and threw it away. This sparked endless phone calls on the house phone throughout the night. His parents would not answer it because they didn't want to deal with him. My mother-in-law said she would tell Danny they were working in the garage as an excuse for not answering the phone. Even his own mother was uneasy about his behavior. I knew this was it. I had to leave the following day. The problem was, it was the middle of October, and my apartment wasn't ready yet. Chloe's school was not ready to accept her either.

I went to the courthouse the following morning to file a restraining order. I chose then to report the attack which took place in March. I knew Danny was coming for me, and I tried that avenue to get help. I was in line and I called him from my new phone I had been hiding. I went ballistic, and made a complete fool of myself there in the courthouse. I screamed at him, said I was leaving, and what I thought of him. I felt like a caged animal that had set herself free.

At first Danny was nice and tried to persuade me. He said, "Come on, it's me. Rebecca, please don't do this. We can work it out." I was persistent and told him to go to hell. Then he flipped, and said, "If you do this, you will die, bitch. I will come at you with full force." I started   shaking because I knew what he was capable of. I hung up and continued my business. He kept calling and calling my phone, and drained the battery. I submitted my paper work for the order and had to wait a couple of hours. My request was denied. It had been too long since the abusive incident, and I couldn't obtain an order on what I thought his response to the divorce would be. I felt defeated and left. I called three of my friends on the way home. I told them I had to leave that night and needed their help.

I got a ride to U-Haul and rented a truck. I was very nervous as I knew I had set the wheels in motion, and couldn't stop. I pulled up in front of the house and accidentally sideswiped the gardener's little truck. I apologetically gave him $200 and asked if we could eliminate getting the insurances involved. I did not have time to deal with another problem. He agreed and took the money. I went in the house and started packing. The whole time I was trying to think of how I would tell Chloe. She had her school Halloween carnival that night. Aunt Carmen knew what was happening and agreed to take her. At 5PM my friends arrived at the house, ready to move me out.

My mother-in-law was in the kitchen, packing up all of my Tupperware and spices. I asked her if she would take care of Chloe, and take her to and from school until I could get her on the first of the month. She said, "Of course I will." It broke my heart knowing I had to leave her. As it was, I was going to stay on a friend's couch until my apartment was ready.

Chloe and Carmen arrived at the house around seven o'clock. She was dressed in her little vampire costume. I took her in her room so I could talk to her alone. I told her the truth. I said her dad and I were going to get a divorce, and we had to move. I apologized to her and said I tried to make it work, but we did not get along. Chloe said, "I understand, mama." I was completely surprised by her response. She had seen Danny bully me and push me around, and knew things weren't going well; however, I did not expect her to take the divorce news so well. She was only seven years old, and did not realize how much her life was about to change.

One thing I left behind when I drove off from the house was my red Nissan Altima. Danny and I had gotten the same car a few months apart. He bought a white one which had both our names on the loan. I bought a red one a month later. I can't recall why, but we put my car in Danny's name only. Although I loved my red car, I was not about to leave a vehicle in his possession that had my name on the loan. In his eyes I drove off with his white car. Later that proved to be a smart choice, as he allowed the red car to get repossessed.

It was midnight when we finished moving everything out. Some of my stuff was in Carmen's garage, some of it was at my friend, Janelle's house, and some of it was at Janelle's mom's house. I stayed the night with one of my girlfriends who helped me move. I put one of my large dresser drawers in the trunk of my car, and kept all my shoes and clothes I would need for a few days. I was in survival mode.

I went to work the following day, and Danny called my business phone non- stop. I had to tell my supervisor what was happening. The institution I worked for was able to block his number. I was humiliated about bringing my personal issues into work, but my supervisor was very understanding. Danny kept calling my cell phone and left a couple of threatening messages. One message said, "What I did to you a couple of months ago will be nothing compared to what I'll do now." He also stated he would try to make it look like I was a drug addict and a prostitute if I tried to go through with the restraining order or divorce. He said he would show everyone the videos he had recorded from my time on-line. I received between 70-95 phone calls a day from him over a several day period.

My mother-in-law called me and was crying. She stated Danny finally returned home and went upstairs where our living quarters were. He saw everything I took and left the house saying he was going to my school that night to kick my ass. I was shaking, and felt unsafe. I walked around my work in a fog. I did my job, but I was dazed. Janelle came up to me and told me to snap out of it and focus. She scolded me and told me not to allow him to break me down. I had a presentation that night at school, and couldn't get out of it. I had two other classmates depending on me to do my part in our project. I had so much on my mind. I was terrified he would come to my school. I was also nervous about my baby being in that house. I felt stronger after talking to Janelle. She always gave me a great deal of support.

After work I went to Carmen's house and told her everything that happened that day. She encouraged me to call WEAVE. This is an organization for victims   of domestic violence. I had never heard of this business, and used them for the wrong recourses. I wanted them to have Danny arrested for harassing me. That was not something the organization was able to do. They provided a safe place to hide, and resources for starting a new life. That was not what I needed. I called the police and told them about Danny's threats. They came to the house, and I had planned to let them listen to his voicemail. When I accessed my voicemail, it had been erased. Danny later told me he figured out my password and deleted them. The police suggested I refrain from going to school that night. I did not have a choice. I had already missed too much school and had to go, or I would not pass the semester. I wasn't going to allow him to take away my future.

I went to school that night and notified them of the threats. The school called the police, and had the parking lot surrounded. I managed to deliver my presentation with my team. I held back the tears and did what I needed to do.

I could not believe this was happening to me. All I wanted was to be free from a terrible marriage. I felt like he was hunting me.

Danny never showed up that night. If he did, he turned around once he saw the police in the parking lot. I went to Carmen's after school, and she told me I could stay with her until my apartment was ready.

That weekend Carmen received a call from my mother-in-law. She told her Danny tried to commit suicide, and was taken to the hospital. I immediately felt angry. I was angry because my daughter was there in the house, and I was also upset he did not succeed. Danny often threatened suicide when things weren't going his way. Carmen's husband, Troy, laughed and said there was my ticket to getting Chloe back.

My in-laws brought her to me that night. It was only a couple of days before she was to start her new school anyway. That evening I received a call from a social worker at the hospital where Danny was taken. She had to call me because of a duty to warn. She stated Danny was locked in the bathroom at the house and said he had taken 40 OxyContin. The police had to break down the door. Danny told them he was going to kill me when they entered the bathroom.

The following morning I went back to the courthouse to obtain my restraining order. I finally had the proof I needed, and the judge granted the order. I also provided the information my daughter gave me. She told me how her daddy told her he was leaving and never coming back because mommy left him. He was trying to prepare her for his suicide, and blame me for it in the process. I don't know why I was surprised, but I could not believe the selfishness that man displayed towards an innocent child. I had to have Danny served with the order within three days. He had been moved to a   locked-down psychiatric facility an hour and half away for a 72-hour hold. I was not allowed to serve him since I was the protected party.

My friend, Linda and I drove to the facility the following day. We got there and told the staff why we needed to access one of their patients. They stated it was unusual for a patient to be served while in lock down. I told them the judge told me he had to be served within a certain time frame, and we could not wait until he was released.

They reluctantly allowed my friend access through a door where many of the patients resided in a day room. Danny was sitting in there and looked like he was in a fog. She handed him the documents and turned around to leave. They had locked her in there with everyone. She panicked and yelled out to open the door. My heart broke for her. They let her out as soon as she asked to leave. I felt terrible for involving my friend in this madness. She was wonderful about the whole situation, and said, "We are done here. Let's go home."

I felt the restraining order was this magic piece of paper which was going to protect me. It did not stop Danny from his ongoing abusive behavior. I moved into my apartment while he was in lock down. So, essentially I had to move twice. Several of my friends got together and picked up my belongings from the various places they were kept. I rented another U-Haul and removed my items from Carmen's garage. I had to move in the evening because I needed everyone's help after work. Again, we finished moving in everything close to midnight. I had also read it was safer to move into an apartment at night so the tenants could not see what you had. My friends told me the second floor was the less likely floor to be robbed, so I chose the second floor apartment. I had to think of everything since I was going to be all alone with my little girl.

I began to cry once I was alone, and everyone had gone home. I cried because I was finally free. I wasn't going to have to listen to constant criticisms, or deal with endless arguments about how I couldn't think correctly. I had waited for this moment for so many years. Then I cried because I had to celebrate my freedom, which was something I deserved to have all along. I was never tearful over the end of my marriage. Once I drove off from that house, I never looked back. Danny had killed any love I felt for him years before that point.

The following day I gave my supervisor at work a copy of the restraining order. Danny had made threats to come to the hospital to attack me, and destroy the car I was driving. He became frustrated when I told him I would not give the car to him. My supervisor told all 60 people in my department to report it if they saw my husband. The hospital was going to announce a code gray if he showed up so security could escort him out. Code gray represented a violent person on the premises. I felt many people looked at me differently after that. There was one dietician in particular who showed judgment on her face whenever I saw her. I felt like trash. How had this become my life? Most of the people I worked with did not know my circumstances, yet chose to look down on me because of my predicament. I became angry all the time. I didn't talk; I yelled. I was so frustrated about everything that had happened and what was continuing to happen to me. Danny never showed up at the hospital or destroyed my car. He only made empty threats to cause a disruption to my life.

It was the night before Christmas Eve, and I was up late building my daughter's Barbie house. Danny kept texting me and asked me to talk to him. He said things like, "You are so fucked up for not talking to me." I called the police, and they came over. I showed him the restraining order, and the officer called Danny from my phone. He told him to stop contacting me or he was going to have to arrest him. Danny persistently stated, "I think I should be allowed to talk to my wife. I have been with her for 16 years." The officer stated there was a restraining order that said differently. Danny left me alone for the rest of the week. After he hung up, the officer told me the order was just a piece of paper, and not really a form of protection. He also stated Danny would have to have his hands around my neck in order to be arrested. The officer advised me to do whatever I needed to do in order to protect myself.

Danny kept finding reasons to call me, and mostly used Chloe as an excuse. He asked if we could get together to discuss everything. He reminded me how we had to be in each other's lives as long as Chloe was a minor. I wanted so desperately for Danny to be a normal individual. I knew I was going to have to deal with him in regards to parenting issues for the next eleven years, and I wanted an amicable divorce. I agreed to meet him at his sister's house. His sister took care of Chloe while we went to dinner. He wanted us to ride in my car (the one he wanted back), and I suggested we take his. We went to dinner and he tried holding my hand. I pulled away from him. He looked hurt and confused. I reminded him we were there to discuss a plan to try to get along for our daughter.

Our discussion went downhill very quickly. He accused me of taking the camera he bought and performing on-line again. I assured him I threw it away and wanted nothing to do with that life anymore. Then he told me to show him my phone. He wanted to go through it to see if there were any names of the guys (customers) I had mentioned on there. I started shaking. I realized he was never going to respect my space and that he still felt he owned me. I told him I wanted to leave. I was physically shaking and started to cry. He became embarrassed as others were watching, so he complied with my request.

We got in the car and started driving. I thought we were going back to his sister's house, but he turned down the wrong street. I asked what he was doing. He said he was going to stay out with me until I agreed to take him back. He pulled into a wooded area not far from his sister's house. I tried to get out of the car, and he pulled the door shut. He held down my hands and started talking to me, and crying. He told me he wanted another chance. He said he wanted to be there for me, in my future, and to see me graduate. He said it was my lips he wanted to kiss. He touched my lips with his fingers. I wanted to vomit. I hated him so much, and didn't want him touching me. I also felt very unsafe as this was false imprisonment. This went on for about a half an hour. I finally started crying uncontrollably. I started screaming with desperation. I wanted that idiot out of my life, and didn't want to feel trapped anymore. Danny became angry and started the car.

He drove back to his sister's house. His sister was waiting outside with Chloe. I got out of the car and he followed me. He tried taking my car keys and said, "Give me back my car." We struggled for a bit, and his sister and brother-in-law told him to leave me alone. I managed to unlock my car, but he grabbed my keys before I made it in. I sat in the car, and Chloe was getting in the back. She yelled and asked us to stop fighting. Danny took the key fob off my key ring, and then threw my keys at me. He flipped me off and drove off in his car. I realized he now had access to unlocking my car. If it wasn't one problem, it was another!

The next day I had to take some time off work to go to the auto mall where we bought the car. I explained the situation to the dealer. They were able to electronically deactivate the key fob for me. They didn't charge me. The guy felt badly for me, and told me to be careful. Dealing with Danny consumed so much of my time between, emotional distress, phone calls and drama. I realize I didn't have to go to dinner with him that night; however, it was my last attempt at trying to be civil with him.

We had to attend a hearing to confirm the length of the order the following week. I had documented and brought a list of all the contact Danny made in violation of the order. Danny mentioned how I had dinner with him. The judge explained the courts become annoyed with the protected party if they are granted protection, and then violate it by going near the perpetrator. I profusely apologized to the court and let them know it was the last time I would try to have contact with Danny, even for parenting issues. The judge was also annoyed with Danny's violations, and scolded him as well. I was granted a five-year restraining order. The only reason Danny was allowed to contact me was about picking up or dropping off our daughter.

Thirteen

The abuse changed me. I had thoughts of having Danny killed before the divorce was final. I didn't want him in my life, and wanted him to suffer. I was also in desperate need for the madness to stop. I thought about offering someone his life insurance money if they killed him. I had a policy on him through my employer, and he was going to be covered until the divorce was final. I never sought out anyone to do the job, but I understood how a person can be driven to such a horrible act. Danny didn't want me; he just didn't want to be left alone. His selfishness was one of the many things about that situation that enraged me. It angered me because I am a good person, and was a very good wife. I cared about him. He only truly cared about himself. The trouble he caused me after I left was entirely fueled by selfishness and stupidity.

I experienced many different thoughts and feelings throughout the course of my relationship with him. We met when I was extremely impressionable, vulnerable, and still trying to develop the person I was to become. I was disconcerted when Danny began to condemn every aspect of my being. Through the years I became exhausted by his criticisms. I felt there was a great deal that was wrong me, but didn't want to be reminded on a daily basis. I often felt frustrated and full of self-doubt. I became stronger after I started going to school, and studied the human mind. Even though I began to realize I was not a deeply flawed individual, it took many years before developing the courage, strength and resources to leave. Those years were terribly frustrating.

I struggled emotionally for the next several years. I was angry, became promiscuous, drank too much, and had difficulty concentrating. In therapy I learned I have post-traumatic stress disorder. This is something I still struggle with, as I have an over-exaggerated startle response, and have continued to have reoccurring nightmares since developing this book.

I obtained my Master's degree in marriage and family therapy in 2014, and I am currently working on my hours to obtain my license as a therapist. I'm also a very good therapist. I'm remarried to a wonderful man who supports me in anything I do. He adores my daughter, and has been a great addition to our family. I finally know what it means to be in a healthy relationship with a man, and can show my daughter what that looks like.

Therapy, time, and learning to love and forgive myself have helped me immensely. The hardest part of my recovery has been letting go of the anger I had towards my ex, and condemning myself for allowing someone to hurt me for so many years. I'm sure many other individuals, who have endured similar circumstances, suffer from the same feelings. In therapy we teach that forgiveness is not for the other person; it's for you. Forgiveness is letting go. I chose to let go, and no longer allow the anger I felt to consume my life. I've also learned that living my life to the fullest, and the way I choose to is the best revenge I can get against him. He will always be the sick person he is, and that is no longer my problem.

My message to anyone who has suffered abuse is to choose to be happy. Don't allow anyone to blame you for not leaving an abusive situation when you "should have." Don't allow the person who hurt you to take up any more space in your head than they already have. Process through your pain, get it out, and give yourself time to heal. Take as much as you need. And most importantly, forgive yourself!

www.ingramcontent.com/pod-product-compliance
Lightning Source LLC
Chambersburg PA
CBHW032146020426
42334CB00016B/1244